Rosendo Chu

CW00471393

NEW APPROACH TO ACUPUNCTURE

DETECTOR OF PATHOLOGICAL ACUPUNCTURE POINTS
THAT DOES NOT TOUCH HUMAN SKIN

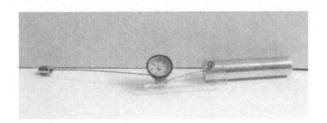

Churion detector

Second edition
2022

Preliminary note

After having carried out different experiments with the detector and having proved its effectiveness, in 1993 I wrote and published in a personal edition the "NEW APPROACH TO ACUPUNCTURE". A very important challenge was that not all people could use the device. They needed to be very sensitive. But since I managed to verify in a simple way the detection of the pathological acupuncture point with a slight modification of the detector, I have been motivated to write a work that is more consistent than the previous one.

INDEX

This law was established by Karl Friedrich Gauss (1777 - 1855), and states that the electric flux or net number of field lines exiting any closed surface is proportional to the net charge enclosed within the surface divided by the electrical permittivity of the medium.It is an alternative procedure for calculating electric fields. It is based on the fact that the fundamental electrostatic force between two-point charges is an inverse square law. Gauss's law is more convenient than Coulomb's law for electric field calculations of highly symmetric charge distributions; it also serves as a guide for understanding more complicated problems.52

INTRODUCTION

This paper is intended for acupuncturists interested in acquiring new knowledge of acupuncture through experimentation and research. A new paradigm does not offer them a discovery about the process of detecting pathological acupuncture points, and a new point-detecting device that does not need to touch the human skin, is very simple and very inexpensive.

Although the text is aimed at acupuncturists, it has a synthesis of what acupuncture is, so that it can be appreciated by a majority of readers and those who are interested in studying acupuncture. As acupuncture is over five thousand years old, it is only in the last two hundred years that new applications have been made; new points discovered, new properties in already known points and the application of electronic devices to detect points, make measurements and treatments. So, a new procedure **to detect pathological points without touching the skin of the human being,** with a simple and inexpensive device, will revolutionize the ancient concept of acupuncture.

I- Acupuncture.

1 - The concept of acupuncture.

Acupuncture is a branch of Traditional Chinese Medicine that has since ancient times a hermetic terminology, a lack of knowledge of the anatomy and pathophysiology of the human being. Thus, for example, its concept of energy has no scientific utility. For this reason, many acupuncture associations refused to use my new acupuncture point detector.

Acupuncture is a diagnostic and therapeutic procedure that consists of inserting very fine metal needles into certain acupuncture points and performing caloric stimulation at these points.

The disease is the result of the imbalance of the vital energy that normally circulates in equilibrium between two forces, but correlated (yin and yang). In a certain number of points in the meridians, the excess or lack of vital energy is found when there is a disease in an organ of the human body.

The diagnosis is made by the acupuncturist by questioning the patient to report their ailments, thus the doctor will review it thoroughly, see and touch as appropriate. Then he will search for the pathological points with various procedures. If he is a Chinese doctor, he will use pulsology, which is the diagnosis by pulses. The Chinese were considered to diagnose not only the total energetic imbalance, but also the type of energy; in addition to determining the meridian where the discomfort was mostly present. The treatment. Once the treatment is done, the use of needles, moxas, massage, herbs, etc. is imposed. The purpose of introducing very fine metal needles into the skin is to regularize the balance of vital energy. When there is an excess of energy in one organ, this excess is transferred to another organ. An example of what is an excess of yin energy, could be that the individual suffers from drowsiness, intense cold, cold edema, etc. And an excess of yang energy could be a feverish state (internal heat), excitation to the point of delirium, insomnia, etc.

2 - Energy.

There are two different visions of energy: One that refers to the Chinese tradition, and the other, simply as vital energy, which we can analyze scientifically from the Western point of view. Understanding acupuncture means knowing traditional Chinese medicine and its philosophy. Thus, energy is a concept that is part of a very complex system and has its own logic. For practical purposes, a synthesis will simply be presented here.

Chinese medicine considers that in man energy circulates permanently and always in the same direction through channels called meridians, where the acupuncture points are located. These meridians connect organs of the human body, these organs not being anatomically united according to western medical science. The hourly cycle of energy is as follows:
The cycle begins with the lungs.

- From 3:00 a.m. to 5:00 a.m. energy passes to the Lungs.
- From 5:00 a.m. to 7:00 a.m. the Large Intestine.
- From 7 a.m. to 9 a.m. the Stomach.
- From 9:00 a.m. to 11:00 a.m. the Spleen - Pancreas.
- At noon it goes to the Heart from 11 am to 1 pm.
- From 1 p.m. to 3 p.m. it passes to the Small Intestine.
- From 3 p.m. to 5 p.m., the Urinary Bladder.
- From 5 p.m. to 7 p.m., the Kidneys.
- From 7:00 p.m. to 9:00 p.m., the Heart Master.
- From 9:00 p.m. to 11:00 p.m., the Three Stoves.
- From 11:00 p.m. to 1:00 a.m. it goes to the Gallbladder.
- From 1:00 a.m. to 3:00 a.m. it goes to the Liver.

Finally, then it would start the cycle again with the Lung

3 - Meridians.

The meridians are the channels through which energy circulates and where the acupuncture points are located. There are different types of meridians according to their function. The most important are the Principal Meridians, whose points are located on the skin. For each side of the body there is a meridian. Each meridian corresponds to an organ, and so for example, for the lungs there is one meridian on the left side and another on the right side; for the heart there are also two meridians, one left and one right. The meridians are connected by accessory channels called Secondary Vessels, which allow the energy to circulate through all the meridians permanently.

To this day, there is no verification of the material existence of the meridians. It is possible that the energy channels are channels of electrical origin, on the basis or principle that when an electric current passes through a conductor, this in turn generates an electric field. As it has been proven that an electric current circulates through the nerves, when electricity circulates, a field is generated. It should be noted that the circulation of electricity through a conductor (a wire) is not the same as how it circulates through the nerves.

Let's see what Professor Li Ding had to say. 1991: "The essential functions of meridian system are 'transport qi and blood, 'to maintain conductivity' and 'to resist invasion of exogenous pathogenic factors" "The meridian theory was not based on empty, but rather on the accumulated observations of many generations of ancient Chinese medical practitioner" "To this day, the meridian theory is the fundamental guiding principle for acupuncture therapy"."

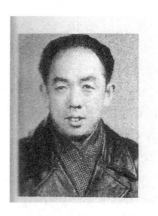

Fig. 1- Professor Li Ding.

4 - Acupuncture points.

The acupuncture point is the point of an energy channel, that when a disorder occurs in an organ or a function, a particular sensitivity occurs: it can be itching or tingling sensation, pain to the touch, dilation of capillaries or inflammation. There are other acupuncture points that are not found in the meridians.

Classification of the points of the main meridians.

Command points.

These are the points that have a specific and important function, capable of modifying the behavior of the meridian or the function of the corresponding organ.

Toning points.

The stimulation of the point allows to increase the amount of energy in the meridian, and the function of the corresponding organ.

Sedation points.

The sedation of the point decreases the energy flow in the meridian, and inhibits the function of the corresponding organ.

Source point.

This is the so-called master point, because depending on how it is stimulated, it will act in the desired direction, that is to say, it can reinforce the tone or disperse the energy of the corresponding organ and regulate its functions.

Passage point.

This is the point that connects each meridian with the source point of its coupled meridian. This point is used to discharge excesses or compensate defects of the energy channel between two neighboring meridians.

Assent points.

It is the point that corresponds to each organ and is located on the bladder meridian, on the back side. It is therefore not on the meridian that acts. This point facilitates a complementary action of regulation of the main point. "It is a point of direct action on the internal organs. It acts by metameric relation, that is to say, through the neurovegetative system. Its general action is sedative" Sussmann, David- 1967.

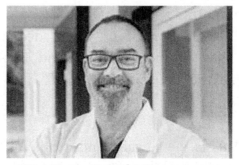

Fig. 2- Dr. David J Sussmann.

Alarm point.

This point is located on the anterior aspect of the trunk and is not located on the same meridian. It becomes sensitive to pain by pressure in case of affection of the corresponding internal organ. Its general action is toning.

Other acupuncture points. There are several groups of acupuncture points that are characterized by their particular action and that the acupuncturist should be aware of these points, they are: a- Point of complementary assent, b- points of reunion, c- Special points, d- The points window to heaven, e- the points of the 5 elements, f- and the master points of the Wonderful Vessels.

II - Localization of acupuncture points.

1- Features of the acupuncture point.

It has been considered that the acupuncture point has a surface of one to two square millimeters and consequently it has been said that in order to practice acupuncture the acupuncturist must be precise in its localization, because if not, the therapy may fail. In this respect I do not agree. Acupuncturists with the experience they have had, they stick the needle without making measurements or calculations. And how do you explain this? I have seen acupuncturists stick the needle as if they were throwing a dart into the patient's body.

What happens is that the acupuncture point has **an electric field** and when the needle is stuck in, a therapeutic effect is produced. Through electrophysiology it has been proven that the points have a weak electrical resistance (Ohms), when a metal needle is stuck near a point, the point is modified by the effect of the electric field.

One of the most common techniques is to touch the meridian suspected of imbalance until the sensitive or painful point is felt. So, a patient says: "It hurts here in the middle of the lung", it turns out that this is a point that has to do with the large intestine.

The point can be perceived as if it were in a hollow, or also a sensation of viscosity. When the point does not have any sensitivity, its location should be considered with the recommendations offered in the acupuncture manuals.

2 - Localization of acupuncture points according to traditional Chinese medicine.

a- Locating the points according to anatomical marks. It has been considered that the references or anatomical marks found on the surface of the skin have a great importance for the location of the points, because the points are found near these anatomical marks.

b - Locate the points according to the proportional division.

This method consists of splitting the different parts of the body in equal parts and each part or division is equivalent to **a cun**, to do this we use some plates that indicate how to perform the division.

c- Measure with the fingers of the hand.

You must measure the distance between the two ends of the folds of the middle finger flexed, this measurement is considered **a cun**, it is also called tsuen which is the Chinese term that means distance. The three recommendations above are not always accurate, so other methods should be used. One of them, very simple, is mentioned by Georges Bau in his book: "Acupuncture - Chinese medicine". "The point is always found in a tiny depression. It is often enough to go over the meridian or the region containing the one you are looking for with a pen. To find that tiny hollow. By resting the pen, the patient feels a pain."

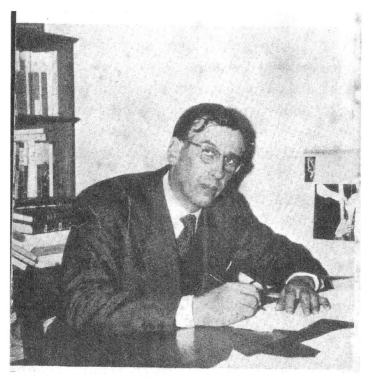

Fig. 3- Dr. Georges Beau.

3 - Acupuncture needles.

At the beginning of acupuncture, fish bones were used, and then iron needles began to be used. These needles are not hollow like hypodermic needles; they are solid and very thin. They are from one centimeter to ten centimeters long, depending on their intended use. An acupuncture needle is two tenths of a millimeter thick, while a needle for injecting liquids is eight tenths.

The use of different metals, according to Soulié de Morant, is due to their intrinsic properties: thus, copper and gold, as toning agents, silver as a dispersant. Iron, steel and platinum would be neutral. Generally, the needles do not produce pain, unless at the moment of the puncture it is a painful point, that happens because not only because they are very thin, but because as long as it is punctured in the acupuncture point or very close to it, no pain will be felt.

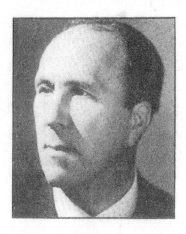

Fig. 4- George Soulié de Morán, 1878- 1955

Other types of needles.
a - The three-edged needle.

This needle has a sharp, triangular-shaped tip. It is used to cause bleeding by pricking gently and superficially.

b - The cutaneous needle.

These are two types of needles and are used to puncture the dermis by hammering.

c - The "Seven Stars" needle.

This instrument is constructed by seven short stainless-steel needles embedded in a round saucer, which has a handle 5 to 6 inches long.

d- The "Plum Blossom" needle.

This instrument consists of five stainless steel needles at the end of the handle which is twelve inches long. The tips of the needles are at the same level and are not very sharp at the tip, this is to avoid producing pain and bleeding.

e - The intradermal needle.

This needle is used for subcutaneous implantation, its application is for stubborn pain and chronic diseases.

There are two types:

The "Chinche" type needle.

These needles are made of stainless steel and silver. They have their origin in a western invention; they are also used in China. These needles are very thin, have a tenth of a millimeter 0, 1 mm and 3 millimeters long. They are introduced perpendicularly to the skin leaving out the head. It is fixed permanently for one or several days. It is generally used for chronic pains of organs. It is widely used in auriculotherapy.

The "Granite" type needle.

This needle is one centimeter long, with a head in the shape of a grain of wheat. It is very suitable for insertion into acupuncture points and painful points in various parts of the body. The needle is inserted with a forceps into the selected point, the handle remains outside, then it is covered with an adhesive tape.

4- Moxibustion in Traditional Chinese Medicine. Moxibustion is a method that treats and prevents diseases by applying heat by means of cones and lit cigars on certain acupuncture points on the human body. The purpose of moxa application is to heat and clear the channels or meridians of obstacles, eliminate cold, dampness and promote organ function.   The   material most commonly used in the manufacture of cones and cigarettes (Moxas) is Artemisia (Artemisis Vulgaris) in the form of fine powder. There are several kinds of moxibustion: with moxa cones, with moxa cigars and thermal needle. Moxibustion with cones can be direct or indirect. Direct moxibustion is when there is scarring (burning) and without scarring. Indirect moxibustion uses an insulating substance such as ginger, garlic or salt. In moxibustion with cigars, the lighted cigar is placed at a distance of one to three centimeters above the acupuncture point. The cigar can be moved intermittently, moving the cigar up and down until the skin turns pink and the patient feels the burning sensation.   The thermal needle procedure is performed after the needle is inserted and the correct acupuncture sensation is obtained, a little moxa is placed on the needle handle and ignited so that the heat is conducted through the needle.

III- Modern acupuncture. New approach to acupuncture.

1 - Introduction.

Modern acupuncture differs from Traditional Chinese Medicine acupuncture in its concept of disease, in the application of new methods of localization of acupuncture points and in new treatments. Thus, we have the electronic detectors of acupuncture points, laser beam therapies, color therapy, sound therapy and finally the new detector of pathological points that does not touch the skin of the human being, does not use batteries and is extremely economical, this is: "The Churion detector".

2- Laser therapy or laserpuncture.

Laser acupuncture is a technique that applies the fundamentals of traditional Chinese acupuncture and replaces needles with a laser beam of low density and without thermal effect. Laser acupuncture has its origin in 1973; it was the Norwegian physician Wilhelm Schjelderup who proposed the use of laser beams to treat acupuncture points, giving rise to the beginning of "modern acupuncture". By 1978 laserpuncture was established and accepted by Traditional Chinese Medicine.

By 2010 acupuncture has been considered world heritage of humanity by UNESCO. It has also been recognized by the World Health Organization as a highly effective alternative means for the treatment of pain.

Laser therapy has many pros: it is painless, unlike needles. It produces no side effects, it is totally safe, it is very easy to apply, and it is compatible with other therapies. Its application is faster than needles.

3 - Colorpuncture.

Colorpuncture is the application of light of different colors on the acupuncture points to transmit light through the meridians to perform treatments. It is considered that the German doctor Peter Mandel was the founder of

Colorpuncture. He studied acupuncture in Hong Kong and India. Later he was researching for 30 years doing clinical observation and discovered how to use colored light applied to the skin at acupuncture points to perform treatments. It is considered that due to the photosensitivity of the body cells, the treatment can be performed with immediate benefits.

4 - The sound therapy.

The sound therapy was created by the jazz musician Fabien Maman of French origin who in 1975 studied acupuncture with the famous Japanese master Nakazano. This therapy is based on the discovery that human blood cells respond to certain sound frequencies, changing shape and color, and the hypothesis that red blood cells and diseased cells can be healed or harmonized with sounds.

Fabien Maman is recognized as the founding father of sound vibration therapy created by him in 1977 and was the initiator of the technique that uses tuning forks and colored lights on acupuncture points, instead of needles.

IV- The detector of pathological acupuncture points of Rosendo Churión.

1- The Churion Detector.

Of all the methods that have been used to detect acupuncture points; perhaps until now there had not been applied a technique that does not touch the skin of the human being when using a mechanical instrument. In acupuncture the insertion of metal needles into the skin, in laserpuncture it is a low intensity laser beam that touches the acupuncture point, in color therapy it is a beam of colored light, in sound therapy it is a sound applied to the point. The procedure of the new detector is based on the use of two metals: aluminum and iron as amplifiers of a bioelectric signal that goes from the patient to the acupuncture physician holding the device; this can happen when an acupuncture point is overloaded with energy; in the opposite case, it can happen that the energy goes from the physician to the patient when an acupuncture point is below the normal level.

For the performance of the use of the new detector it is indispensable that the acupuncturist physician is in good health conditions. Otherwise, if a part of the body is sick and requires energy, then the patient's energy may flow to the sick part of the practitioner's body. Here a false diagnosis could occur, that the acupuncturist has drawn energy from a point that was not overloaded and as a result the practitioner felt the signal on the handle of the device.

2 - Modern dowsing and acupuncture.

The new procedure should not be confused with modern dowsing which corresponds to a technique of mental power using rods, a pendulum or an aurameter in order to obtain an answer to a question asked to the unconscious mind of the dowsing operator. With the "Churion Detector" the acupuncturist begins to pass the apparatus very close to the patient's skin; in this case the acupuncturist is not asking himself any question that requires an immediate answer; if the acupuncturist does not receive a signal, nor does the patient, this should indicate that it is not a pathological point. The acupuncturist should then perform his or her search in another area of the meridian.

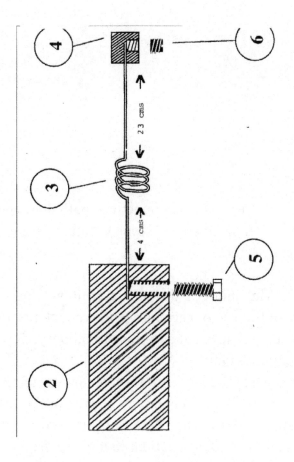

Fig. 5- The first Churion Detector.

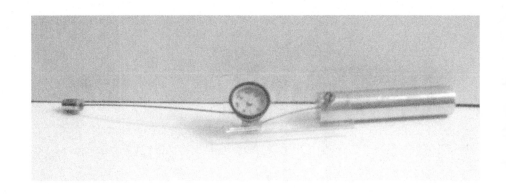

Fig. 6 - The new acupuncture pathology point detector that does not touch human skin: the Churion Detector.

The modern dowsing technique does not require the use of certain types of metal, nor does it require that the device be placed very close to the patient's skin.
The dowser expects to receive an unconscious neuromuscular response to a previously asked question. With the "Churion Detector" if a physician is told by a patient that he has pain in the kidneys, the physician will place the new detector on the kidney meridian points and check for pathology, which can be checked by performing an echosonogram or a urine test. As can be seen, it works with prior information. In the case of dowsing, the information is generally very scarce.

The Churion Detector is not for dowsing, although it may happen that a person wants to use it and it works. Let's see an example: it is as if a person were to use a scalpel to cut a piece of beef.

3 - Acupuncture.

Acupuncture has five thousand years of empirical experience in China and almost a century of scientific verification. Acupuncture is the introduction of metallic needles and caloric stimulation at points connected to energy lines that are the twelve meridians.   The energy is produced by the viscera and organs and circulates through all the meridians. When a blockage of energy occurs in a meridian, pain, swelling, congestion of capillaries, etc. will occur. When a disease occurs, the acupuncturist will try to find out if there is any abnormality in some meridian points.Acupuncture points are characterized by a very low electrical resistance. It was Niboyet, J.E.H who discovered in 1951 that acupuncture points have a lower resistance to the passage of direct current (DC). From this discovery, devices to detect acupuncture points began to be manufactured. The acupuncturist who knows the acupuncture points from experience can use the point detector to verify their existence, if not to perform a measurement and even a treatment without needles, if the device allows it.   "One criticism that has been made of electrical detection is that more points appear than classically described, a fact that shows that the integument (skin) does not present a homogeneous structure and that the points of least resistance constitute a physiological phenomenon hitherto unknown"- Sussmann, David.J.-1967.

This phenomenon is understood because in all parts of the body there are nerves, and these conduct electrical energy. A new scientific acupuncture should emerge in the future taking into account this phenomenon.

V-Brief history of the detector. Chronology of events.

1- Since 1983 I was dedicated to the manufacture of dowsing instruments that I made for sale, and also attended several times to acupuncture courses that were held at the Venezuelan Institute of Natural Medicine, either to learn acupuncture, but to sell acupuncture books, alternative medicines and dowsing devices. So out of curiosity I began to experiment with the doctors who attended the acupuncture courses, when I tried to capture the aura with the aurameter I felt a slight electric current in the handle I was holding. I asked other doctors to try the aurameter and see if they felt anything. Some did, some did not. I then went on to study acupuncture in depth and to continue experimenting with the device.

Finally, I came to see that it detected the pathological points of the human being, either because they had an excessive accumulated energy, or because they were very weak in energy.

2- Patent application in 1985 granted on December 21, 1993.

On December 21, 1993 I introduced before the Ministry of Development the patent application of invention, in that opportunity I used the aurameter, which was an apparatus to use it in Modern Dowsing. The cavity in the handle is only useful in dowsing, but it was left that way in case the cavity could be needed later to make improvements, but it did not happen that way.

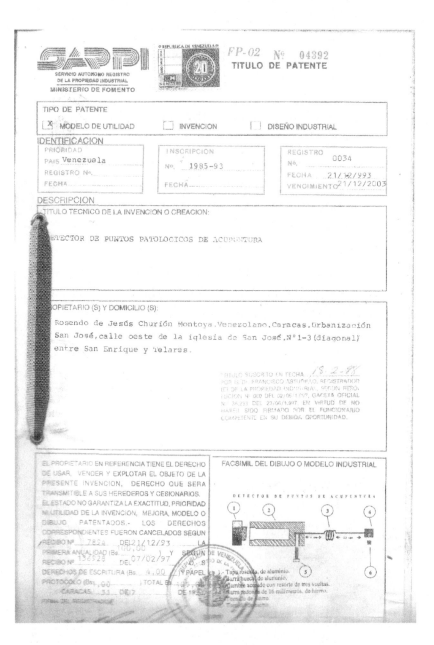

Fig. 7- Invention patent document.

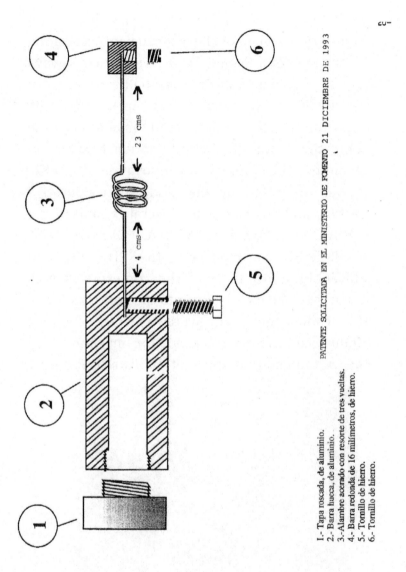

PATENTE SOLICITADA EN EL MINISTERIO DE FOMENTO 21 DICIEMBRE DE 1993

1.- Tapa roscada, de aluminio.
2.- Barra hueca, de aluminio.
3.-Alambre acerado con resorte de tres vueltas.
4.- Barra redonda de 16 milímetros, de hierro.
5.- Tornillo de hierro.
6.- Tornillo de hierro.

Fig. 8- The first detector of pathological
acupuncture points.

2- On May 6, 1984 I received the diploma of Honorary Member of the Venezuelan Association of Acupuncture. Signed by Dr. Teodórico Sawaya López - President and Dr. Piero Gallo. Professor of the U.C.V. - Secretary. 3- In April 1995, the opportunity arose to present my invention to the competition for the Third National Salon of Inventions, Discoveries and Innovations EUREKA. It was organized by the: Asociación Educativa Vértice, and sponsored by several organizations: CONICIT, FUNDACIÓN SIVENSA, PDVSA, CANTV, MINISTERIO DE FOMENTO (SARPI), CVG, and CERVECERÍA POLAR. The contest was held in Caracas - Venezuela. Prior to the participation of the contestants, we were given a course: "Industrial Property Workshop for Innovators". By the Autonomous Service of Industrial Property

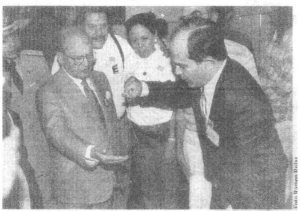

El presidente encargado, doctor Ramón Escovar Salom, se somete a experimentación con un aparato que sirve para la digitoacupuntura.

Registry.

Fig. 9 - Photo from the newspaper EL NUEVO PAÍS-
Monday, May 8, 1995- page 27.

In the photo Eng. Simón Parisca President of
EUREKA and Mrs. María Corina Parisca de
Machado. The president in charge Dr. Ramón
Escobar Salom is submitted by Rosendo Churión
with the acupuncture points detector.

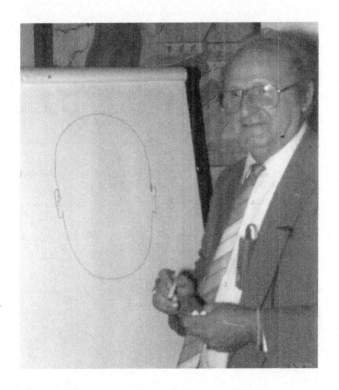

Fig. 10 - Dr. Teodórico Sawaya López in his
acupuncture class.
July 21, 1921 - December 1, 2013.

INSTITUTO VENEZOLANO DE MEDICINA NATURAL

Lic.Rosendo Churión.
Presente.-   Caracas,23 de febrero de 1995.

Estimado licenciado:

Con motivo de la presentación de su invento "el detector de puntos patológicos de acupuntura" en el "Salón Eureka",queremos hacer público que hemos sido testigo de como el aparato lo han utilizado médicos graduados en los cursos de acupuntura,con unas simples instrucciones y con mucho éxito.

Está demostrado así que no se reuiere de una sensibilidad especial.Asi mismo reconocemos que el detector por usted inventa do es útil para detectar los tuntos patológicos de acupuntura en el ser humano,como también los niveles de energía en el estado de salud.

Estamos a la disposición de cualquier jurado que esté interesado en la demostración de su utilidad o algun medio de comunicación social.El licenciado Rosendo Churión es miembro honorario de nuestra institución desde el 12 de abril de 1984,por eso nos complace que un miembro nuestro se dedique a la investigación con tan buenos resul tados.Sirva nuestro testimonio como un reconocimiento para que tenga éxito en la exposición "Salón Eureka"

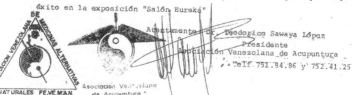

Atentamente Dr. Teodorico Sawaya López
Presidente
Asociación Venezolana de Acupuntura
Telf. 751.94.86 y 752.41.25

Fig. 11 - Letter from the Venezuelan Institute of Natural Medicine.

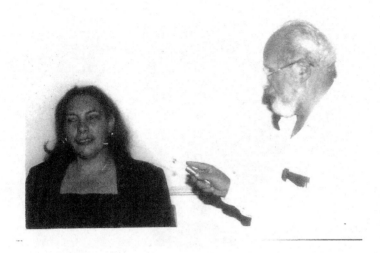

Fig. 12 - Dr. Teodórico Sawaya López using the detector.

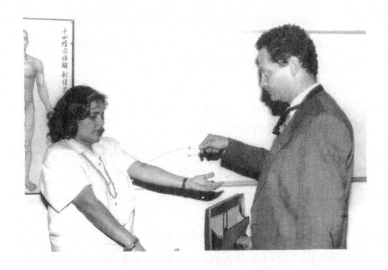

Fig.13 - Dr. Edgar Gómez Gómez -U.C. V, using the detector.

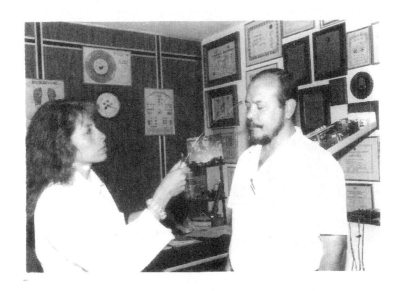

Fig. 14 - Dr. Frida Eli Tapia using the detector.

4- II Congress of Popular Technology. 1995.
Certified as a speaker, title of the paper: "New Approach to Acupuncture".
Lisandro Alvarado University.
President Rector. José Bethelmy.
Vice-president: Dr. Francisco Mieres.
Executive Secretary: Economist José Furiati.
Place: Barquisimeto. Lara State - Venezuela.
Date: July 6, 7 and 8, 1995.

5 -VI International Congress of the Spanish-American Acupuncture Association, Beijing - 84.:
Venezuela-La Guaira. Macuto Sheraton Hotel.
Date: April 1997. Organized by: Nei Jing School of Maracay. Aragua State. Doctors: Jesús Velásquez and Juan José Sánchez.   In this congress I made

the presentation of the invention "Detector of pathological acupuncture points" and it was tested with several doctors attending this congress. The result was that a group of acupuncture doctors who had come from Mexico asked me to borrow the detector for them to practice in the hotel during the breaks. The next day they bought the entire stock of detectors from me. The bad news

The bad news is that we agreed to keep in touch by mail, but I wrote to them several times and got no response. A few months later a photograph appeared with the discovery of a large number of large and small mailing envelopes that never arrived at their destination because those

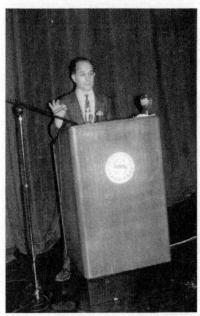

who administered the mail kept the money.

Fig. 15 - Rosendo Churión giving a brief
presentation on the detector.

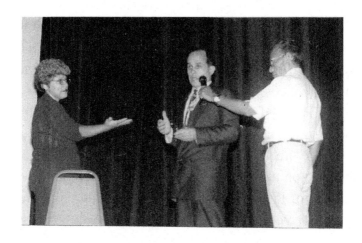

Fig.16 - Rosendo Churión explaining the use of the
detector, Dr. Capistrán Alvarado from Mexico
holds the microphone for him.

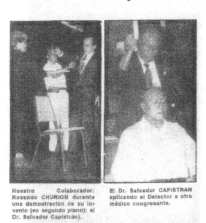

Nuestro   Colaborador:
Rosendo CHURION durante
una demostración de su invento (en segundo plano): el
Dr. Salvador Capistrán).

El Dr. Salvador CAPISTRAN
aplicando el Detector a otro
médico congresante.

Fig. 17- Photographs published in the March 1997
issue of Cábala Magazine.

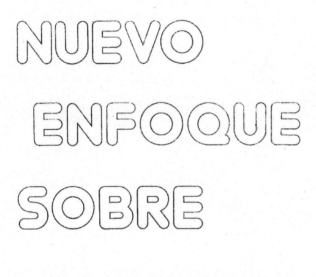

NUEVO

ENFOQUE

SOBRE

ACUPUNTURA

ROSENDO CHURIÓN

Fig. 18 – Independent publishing of the
acupuncture point detector.
Caracas - 1993.

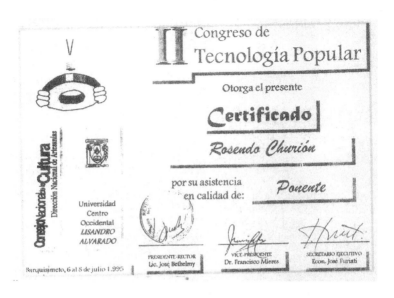

Fig. 19- Speaker's Diploma at the II Congress of Popular Technology.

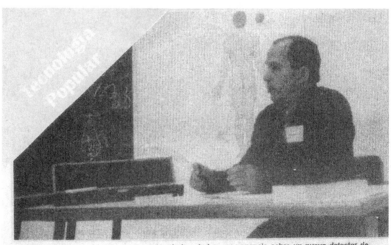

Rosendo Churión ante profesionales de la salud en su ponencia sobre un nuevo detector de puntos de acupuntura.

Fig. 20 - Rosendo Churión while giving his lecture on acupuncture.

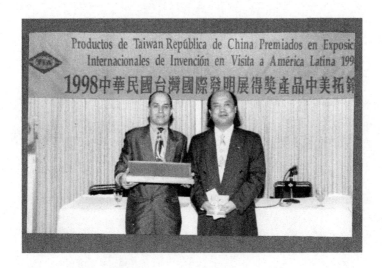

Fig. 21- Rosendo Churion with his acupuncture point detector, accompanied by Mr. Pingchao.

7- Exhibition of Inventions made in Taiwan - Republic of China. 1998.

In this exhibition I had the opportunity to present my invention: "The detector of pathological points of acupuncture that does not touch the skin of the human being". There I presented my invention to the president of the Taiwan Inventors Association and he presented me with one of his own inventions (A pen that has many utilities), organized by the Economic and Cultural Office of Taipei. Place: Caracas -

Venezuela. Caracas Hilton Hotel. Ceiba and Apamate Rooms. Date: February 10, 1998.

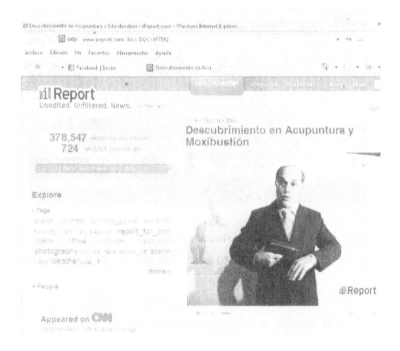

Fig. 22 - New discovery of Acupuncture and Moxibustion. Rosendo Churión explaining how moxas can be replaced by a tin soldering gun. This video was on the Internet for a short time because it seems that it did not have the interest of the public.

VI - The emergence of the pathological acupuncture point detector.

1-Introduction.

As you have seen and read what has happened with the "Acupuncture pathological point detector that does not touch human skin" which was not successful due to many problems. It is now when the main problem I consider it solved. It had happened that a large majority of users of the detector did not have the sensitivity to receive the signal, so with the new model of detector, the user can test its sensitivity, and not only that, with the passage of time the user will increase its sensitivity.

2- Description of the Churion Detector.

The device is made of a solid round aluminum bar, with an extension of 10 centimeters long and with a diameter of 22 millimeters (thickness). At one end of the round bar is inserted a nickel-plated steel wire, with a thickness of 1.5 mm and a length of 20 cm. The steel wire is supported by a screw.

The steel wire at the base has a spring form (six turns which is the coil) and at the other end of the wire there is a round iron rod, which is held to the wire by a screw. The diameter is 9.3 mm (thickness) and the length is 16 mm.

VII - The theory of operation of the "Churion Detector".

a- Basic concepts.

The human being functions in its totality with the electric current that moves through the nerves. Just as it has been proven that when an electric current passes through a conductor (Hans Christian Oersted. 1777-1851) an electric field is generated and Michael Faraday (1791-1867) in 1831 traced the magnetic field around a conductor through which an electric current circulates and discovered electromagnetic induction. Electromagnetic induction is the process by which a current can be induced by a change in the magnetic field. He thus demonstrated the induction of one electric current by another, and induced the concept of lines of force, to represent magnetic fields.

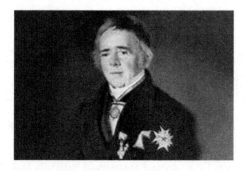

Fig. 23 - Hans Christian Oersted. 1777-185.

Faraday's Law.

Faraday's Law states that, whenever the magnetic field flux through the area bounded by a closed conducting loop (coil) changes, an electromotive force is produced in the loop. The fem produced is given by: $\xi = -d\emptyset/dt$ where $\emptyset = \int B ds$ is the flux of the magnetic field through the area. $\emptyset$ is called the magnetic flux.

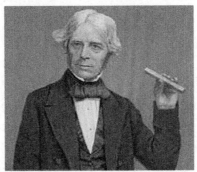

Fig. 24 - Michael Faraday. (1791-1867)

Faraday-Lenz Law.

Faraday's Law was completed with Lenz's Law (Heinrich Friedrich Emil Lenz (1804-1865).

Lenz's law is a consequence of the principle of conservation of energy applied to electromagnetic induction. It was formulated by Heinrich Lenz in 1833. While Faraday's law tells us the magnitude of the EMF produced, Lenz's law tells us in which direction the current flows, and states that the direction is always such that it opposes the flux change that produces it. This means that every magnetic field generated by an induced current goes in the opposite direction to the change in the original field.

Ampère's law.

André Marie Ampère (1775-1836). In 1820 he studied the relationship between magnetism and electricity. He discovered that the direction taken by the needle of a compass depends on the direction of the electric current circulating near the compass. In 1827 he formulated the theory of electromagnetism. Ampère's law explains that the circulation of magnetic field strength in a closed boundary is equal to the current flowing in that boundary. The magnetic field is an angular field with a circular shape, whose lines enclose the current. The direction of the field at a point is tangential to the circle enclosing the current. The magnetic field decreases inversely with the distance from the conductor.

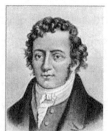

Fig. 25- André Marie Ampère (1775-1836).

Coulomb's Law.

Charles-Augustin de Coulomb (1736-1806-French). In 1789 he published the results of his experiments and established quantitatively the force produced between two electric charges that attract or repel each other. This force is directly proportional to the product of the charges and inversely proportional to the distance. In his honor it was called coulomb or coulomb, as it is known, the unit of measurement of electric charges.

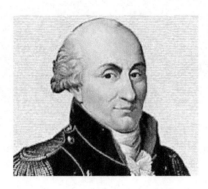

Fig. 26- Charles- Agustín de Coulomb. (1736-1806 French).

Gauss's Law of Magnetism.

This law was established by Karl Friedrich Gauss (1777 - 1855), and states that the electric flux or net number of field lines exiting any closed surface is proportional to the net charge enclosed within the surface divided by the electrical permittivity of the medium. It is an alternative procedure for calculating electric fields. It is based on the fact that the fundamental electrostatic force between two-point charges is an inverse square law. Gauss's law is more convenient than Coulomb's law for electric field calculations of highly symmetric charge distributions; it also serves as a guide for understanding more complicated problems.

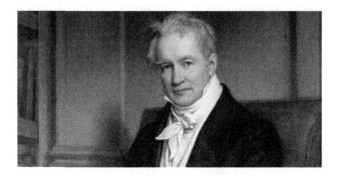

Fig. 27- Friedrich Gauss. (1777 – 1855)

Static electricity.

Static electricity is a phenomenon of surfaces and is generated when two or more bodies come into contact with each other. Static electricity is a non-moving electric charge that accumulates on a material, whether it is a conductor or an insulator, and is abruptly released when it comes into contact with another conductive material. When contact or friction occurs, the materials become positively or negatively charged. The magnitude and polarity of the charge depend on several factors: the material (metals, human skin), temperature, humidity, pressure, and the speed of separation.

Churion's Law.

"When a conductor held by a hand that is constituted by two metals (Iron and aluminum) when approaching the iron to the electric field of a pathological acupuncture point, if the point has less electric charge, an electric charge will pass from the aluminum part towards the iron part and the electric charge will pass to the point modifying it. If the point the pathological acupuncture point has a greater amount of electric charge, an electric charge will pass through the iron and aluminum toward the hand of the one holding the conductor, the point is modified."   Seen in another way this law is as follows: "The strength of the energy increases directly proportional to the reduction of the distance from the tip of the detector, and decreases inversely proportional to the increase of the distance from the tip of the apparatus".

In this Law electric charges attract; in Coulomb's Law they attract or repel.

Electric charge.

All matter is made up of atoms that have equal numbers of electrons (negatively charged) and protons (positively charged). Atoms and molecules can be electrically charged and this is what influences how they attract or repel each other and how matter is formed.

Electric current.

The electric current is formed by charged particles (positive or negative) that flow through a conductor that can be a copper wire, iron, aluminum, the nerves of a human being, etc. The passage of current can be measured in amperes, or milliamperes (A). Electric current is the circulation of electricity moving through conductors in a closed circuit. There are great quantities of types of current, in our work we are only going to refer to two:

Types of electric current.
Alternating current (A.C.)

The alternating current is characterized because the current flow alternates or changes in one direction and in another (the opposite). Direct or direct current (C.D). The direct or direct current is characterized because the electrons always move in the same direction through the conductor and the current intensity is constant.

The volt.

The volt is perhaps the best-known unit of measurement of electricity, because anyone has had to use a battery for the computer, a battery for the cell phone, the car battery, etc. To measure volts, a voltmeter is used, the two tips must be connected or touch both poles (positive and negative). To measure current, an amperemeter is used but the tips of the amperemeter must be placed on a single conductor. Thus, the volt is the potential difference measured at the two points of a two-conductor cable. Direct current (D.C.) can be positive or negative.

The electric field.

The electric field is the area or spatial zone where electric charges, which can be positive or negative and are related in a given space limit, are located. The electric field itself is not measurable, but what is measured is the effect generated by the electric charges within it. When a body moves in the electric field of another, the forces of attraction or repulsion become apparent. The electric field has magnitude and direction; it is an area where the line of force exists. It is therefore a vector quantity. The symbol E expresses the electric field and is measured in Newton/coulomb.

The magnetic field.

The space where its poles have a force of attraction or repulsion is the magnetic field. The magnetic field also induces when electric charges move in space or in an electric conductor. Magnetic field lines are a vector quantity because they have magnitude and direction. The symbol B corresponds to the magnetic field, and is measured in Tesla or Newton per meter.

Differences between electric field and magnetic field.

1- The main difference between electric field and magnetic field is that the electric field is induced around the static charge particle which is either negative or positive; while the magnetic field is produced around the poles (North pole and South pole) of the magnet.

2- The electric field is produced by a unit of polar charge, either by a positive or negative charge; while in the magnetic field it is produced by two poles (the North Pole and the South Pole).

3- The electric field lines do not form a loop, while the magnetic field lines form a closed loop.

4- The electric field is directly proportional to the flux, while the magnetic field strength depends on the number of field lines produced.

5- In an electric field, equal charges repel and different charges attract; while in a magnetic field equal poles repel and different poles attract.

6- Electric fields are induced by a single charge, either positive or negative. While magnetic fields induce with the two poles (north and south).

7- The intensity of the electric field is expressed with the symbol E, while the intensity of the magnetic field is expressed as B.

8- Electric field lines are measured in two dimensions, while magnetic field lines are measured in three dimensions.

9- The electric field line can do work, that is, the velocity and direction of the charge change; whereas in the magnetic field it cannot do work because the direction of the charge changes, but the velocity of the particles remains constant.

b- The materials of which the Churion Detector is made".

The use of aluminum and iron was the consequence of having used the apparatus when experimenting with Modern Radiesthesia practices and finding out if the human aura could be detected physically. When a magnetic flux was detected in the handle of the device, the pathological acupuncture points began to be investigated.   It was found that many users received the signal in the handle. Much   later, when the percentage of electrical conductivity of the materials (iron and aluminum) was investigated, it was found that aluminum is more electrically conductive than iron. Aluminum has a conductivity percentage of 61% and iron 17%. Aluminum is a paramagnetic material, which means that it has the property of being easily magnetized. Aluminum is considered to be a material that is easily charged with static electricity.

c- Acupuncture meridians.

Until today there is no scientific definition of what acupuncture meridians are. We know that in the human body information travels through the cells that constitute the nerves, and that this conduct electricity. Although it has been proven that electricity exists in the human body and that it is conducted by nerves, it cannot be equated or equated to an electrical conductor such as a wire because it has been proven to have other characteristics. There is a hypothesis based on the evidence of the transmission of information by biophotons that was developed by the physicist Fritz Albert Popp. (1938- 2018), that meridians could be like fiber optic cables that carry large amounts of bioinformation in the form of biophotons and with the function, among others, of improving the regulation and organization of biological systems.

The spectral distribution of biophotons covers the range from 200 to 800 nanometers. The presence of infrared radiation belonging to the wide wavelength range of biophotons in structures of the human body was first demonstrated by Dr. Fritz Albert Popp and Dr. Klaus Peter Schlebusch of Germany to be identical to the meridian system described by Chinese acupuncture.

d- The operation of the "Churion Detector".

The Churion Detector is a device that works with the electricity of the user (the acupuncturist) and the electricity of the patient. When the practitioner holds the detector by the handle, it is charged with static electricity and when the acupuncturist places the device on a pathological acupuncture point about four to five millimeters from the point, an electrical charge is produced that can go in the direction of the acupuncturist and felt in the handle, in this case it happens because the pathological point is charged with energy. If the opposite happens, that the pathological point is weakened, i.e., devoid of energy, then static electricity will flow from the handle to the patient. In this case the patient may feel a slight tingling sensation. As most human beings were not sensitive when using the detector (I am referring to the device patented a long time ago). That is why the new detector comes with a compass, which when the tip of the detector is placed on a pathological point, the needle will move in a direction that will indicate whether the pathological point emitted some energy or received it, i.e., the passage of an electric current has occurred. By slightly moving the handle of the detector, electrical charges can be induced to stimulate the pathological point devoid of energy.

The Churion Detector has a compass

installed on the coil, so that when the acupuncturist places the tip of the device near the acupuncture point the needle should move in one direction. This phenomenon was discovered by André Marie Ampère in 1820 who proved that the direction taken by the compass needle depends on the direction of the electric current circulating nearby, hence the so-called Ampere's Rule.

The operation of the detector. What happens between the tip of the Churion Detector and the acupuncture point that does not come into contact, but if they influence each other is by electrostatic induction which is the movement of an electric charge that occurs between both: the tip of the detector and the acupuncture point. How it works. When the acupuncture point is negatively charged and an excess of electrons occurs, this charge tends to pass to the detector; if the detector is negatively charged, the negative charge will pass to the acupuncture point which is in positive, it is in deficiency. Whenever the detector tip approaches an acupuncture point, it modifies the acupuncture point. If the acupuncture point was negative, it will become positive; and if the acupuncture point was positive, it will become negative. The capacity of an object (the detector and the acupuncture point) is the facility they have to hold an electric charge. If two objects of different capacities such as the detector and the acupuncture point are charged with the same amount of electricity, the charge will be more concentrated in the acupuncture point because it has a lower capacity. Thus, the pressure developed by the electricity in the part of smaller capacity (the points) will be of a greater power of repulsion of the charges of the same sign (- and -) and (+ and +) than that of the Churion Detector.

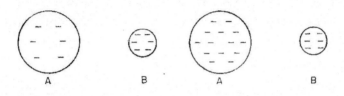

Fig. 28- The electrostatic capacity in objects.
The letter A corresponds to the Churion Detector and the letter B corresponds to the acupuncture point.

WARNING: The device should not be placed near electronic devices such as a television, electric stove, or computers, so as not to cause interference or electric shock. It should not be held by hand and kept in a field during thunderstorm weather to avoid attracting lightning. It should be avoided that children take it as a toy.

e- Human bioelectricity.

In order to have a broader knowledge about the Churion Detector we must be very clear about how electricity works in the human body. This is very important because the Churion Detector works with the electricity of the user of the device and the electricity that exists in the patient's body.

Human bioelectricity is the study of the mechanisms of electrical flow in the human body: how electricity is produced in the human body and how it moves inside the body and the functions it performs.

Difference between physical electricity and human electricity. Let's call physical electricity the electricity used in homes, factories and all kinds of electronic devices. Human electricity is the electricity that exists in the human body and is transmitted by nerves throughout the human body to perform all the functions that keep the body healthy. Physical electricity occurs by the movement of electrons through metal conductors. Human electricity is produced by the flow of charged ions between different cells.

Human skin. The human skin, which is precisely where the tip of the Churion Detector is going to approach, has a constant bioelectrical activity and its electrical conduction capacity varies according to the degree of hydration, the level of stress and the pathological condition of the patient. Its electrical potential is of the order of micro volts (mV). Dry skin has a high resistance estimated at 4,000 ohms 4 K. Ohm. When the skin is wet, it is reduced to 1,500 ohms 1.5 K Ohm. The flow of physical electric current passing through a conductor or several can be measured scientifically with a large number of measures and perform calculations of the magnitudes that are necessary; while the flow of human electricity occurs by electrical and chemical stimuli, and this occurs not only in nerve cells (Neurons) also in muscle cells. It has been proven that electrical stimuli can travel throughout the human body in less than a second, so it can produce a muscle contraction, or release of hormones to regulate body functions, etc.

f- What is electrolysis?

Michael Faraday investigated electrolysis and in 1834 established two laws that bear his name: Faraday's Laws or Laws of Electrolysis are formulas that express quantitatively the quantities deposited on the electrodes.

1- Faraday's law of electrolysis.

Faraday's first law explains the direct relationship between mass, time, intensity and the intrinsic characteristics of the solution, the tissue in dysfunction, in this case. Its statement is:

63

"M=k Q. The mass of the substances deposited or released at each electrode is directly proportional to the electric charge (Q), the electric charge being the product of intensity times time." M = k I t

Where k would be the electrochemical equivalent of the substance Time (t) is a fundamental value in electrolysis. Otherwise, we can read it as follows:

The amount of mass deposited on an electrode is proportional to the amount of electricity that has flowed through the electrode: mass released = K (Constant) times Q times I times T.

K equals 96500 coulombs (Faraday's constant).

Q is equivalent to the charge measured in coulombs.

I is equivalent the current measured in amperes.

T is equivalent time measured in seconds.

2-Faraday's law of electrolysis.

The mass of a substance altered at an electrode during electrolysis is directly proportional to the amount of electricity transferred to this electrode. The amount of electricity refers to the amount of electric charge, which is generally measured in coulombs. For a given amount of electricity (electric charge), the mass of an elemental material altered at an electrode is directly proportional to the equivalent weight of the element. The equivalent weight of a substance is its molar mass divided by its oxidation number, which depends on the reaction taking place in the material. In other words, we can read it as follows:

The amount of deposited mass of an element on an electrode is proportional to its equivalent weight (atomic weight divided by its oxidation number): where the Mass given off = K = 96500 coulombs (Faraday's constant) times the atomic weight divided by the oxidation number.

3rd Faraday's Law of Electrolysis:
The amount of electricity that is necessary for an equivalent gram of an element to be deposited is F = 96500 coulombs (Faraday's constant). As 1 equivalent gram is equal to the atomic weight / oxidation number in grams: mass released = I x T times (atomic weight / oxidation number) divided by 96500.

I Equivalent to the current intensity measured in amperes.
T Equivalent to the time measured in seconds.

The production of electricity in the human body is due to the flow of charged ions between different cells. The process or mechanism is called the "sodium-potassium gate". In order for communication to occur between cells in the human body, this gate is opened, and then sodium and potassium ions can move freely in and out of the cell. The negatively charged potassium leaves the cell, and the positively charged sodium ions enter the cell and electricity is produced. After this occurs, it continues to the next cell, then to the next cell, and so the process continues, until the process of sending messages ceases.

Electrical stimuli can produce a muscle contraction or cause a release of hormones to regulate body functions. In this process in the human body an amount of 10 to 100 milli volts is generated. The measurement of electrical currents is used for analysis with electrocardiograms and encephalograms to measure the electrical potentials of organs such as the heart and brain. Today the application of electrolysis is used for therapeutic purposes; this technique uses devices to promote some physical-chemical changes in a tissue, which induces its recovery in a natural way after the application of electrolysis. It consists of applying a galvanic current through a needle similar to the one used in acupuncture, in the injured area, in order to provoke a chemical reaction that breaks the tissue and produce the current.

VIII - How to make a diagnosis and treatment.

1-Who can use the Churion Detector?

a- It is essential that the user has sufficient knowledge of acupuncture.

b- It is important that the acupuncture practitioner is in good health, so that there is no misdiagnosis of a pathology, because the detector works with the electricity of the body of the practitioner and the patient.

c- It is not necessary a special condition of the user, but it is advisable to practice training and make some checks.

d- When it is a sick person who wants to give himself the treatment, if he is in conditions checked by the acupuncturist doctor, he should give the instructions to the patient.

2- Diagnosis.

The physician must treat the patient as a whole, not just cure a disease. He must start with the interrogation, then the inspection, the examination of the pulses and the abdominal palpation which is a Japanese method known since the year 1700 (Okabe and Kinoshita), and finally perform any test that modern medicine uses, such as ultrasonography, blood and urine tests, etc.

After having performed all the necessary

examinations on the patient, the acupuncturist should study the meridian corresponding to the symptoms presented by the patient starting with the source point, and then, if necessary, investigate the other points. - To make the diagnosis with the Churion Detector, the acupuncturist must take into account the time cycle of the energy.

3- Treatment.

In Traditional Chinese Medicine, the purpose of the treatment is to restore the energetic balance; for this purpose, needles, moxas, massages, acupressure, infusions, herbal decoctions, etc. are used. The Churion Detector cannot replace needles when several needles are to be used in a treatment. It is possible to experiment with a point where it is necessary to increase or decrease the energy of a meridian. The acupuncturist should then tightly grip the handle of the device and bring the tip to about three millimeters of proximity. The time may vary according to the pathology of the patient. It can be from one to three minutes. If the acupuncturist needs to perform a very large energy discharge, he/she should use the other hand to touch a metallic object that makes contact with the earth. If it is a question of charging a pathological point with energy, the acupuncturist should bring the tip of the detector closer and make the tip move slightly over the point; the time will be decided by the acupuncturist according to the patient's condition.

4- The usefulness and characteristics of the Churion Detector.

a - Its main characteristic is that the Churion Detector is designed to detect pathological acupuncture points accurately when the tip of the device is placed near the acupuncture point.

b- It is useful for diagnosing diseases and checking the health status of the human being. If no pathological point is detected when checking all the meridians, it should be presumed that the person is in good health.

c- The Churion Detector can be used by the acupuncture physician for diagnosis and treatment, but it can also be used on your own body. Either to relieve pain while waiting for the result of the administration of a remedy, an analgesic.

d- If a patient does not want to be touched on the skin, either because he has a recent wound, the Churion Detector can be very useful.

e- In case of an emergency, a pathological point on a meridian, either an excess of energy or a deficiency, can be quickly detected. Then the acupuncturist can analyze the rest of the symptoms depending on the case.

f- As it is a device that does not use electric batteries, it is quite practical because it can be taken anywhere in the country.

g- The Churion Detector is of economical manufacture because it does not have electronic components.

IX - Moxibustion. New method.

Moxibustion is a procedure of caloric stimulation of the acupuncture point, in many occasions it can be more effective than needles. If using the Churion Detector on a point does not produce a rapid or desired response, it is recommended to use caloric stimulation of the point; otherwise, use needles. Traditional Chinese acupuncture uses mugwort cones with incense sticks or mugwort cigarettes, which after being lit are placed near the point. Now the new procedure in moxibustion is to use a tin soldering iron, those that are used to repair electronic devices. A soldering iron can be used, but it takes a long time to heat up, so I recommend the use of a soldering gun, just press the switch on the gun to produce heat immediately. When placed on the acupuncture point, the patient should be asked to report what kind of sensation he/she feels, when he/she says that he/she feels a burning sensation, the tip of the soldering iron should be removed. The procedure can then be repeated 3 to 5 times.

Caloric stimulation can be performed on 4 to 6 points.

X- Other types of acupuncture.

In addition to Chinese acupuncture there are two types of acupuncture: auricular acupuncture or ear acupuncture and manopuncture which is hand acupuncture. Both use one part of the body to influence the whole body.

1- Korean manopuncture.

Manopuncture is known as Koryo Sooji Chim - Korean acupuncture. This technique is a form of acupuncture and moxibustion that affects the entire human body with only treatment on the hands. The inventor of the system was Dr. Yoo Tae Woo in Korea, and then started in Japan in 1978; it is already spread all over the world.

The technique of manopuncture has been widely accepted for its effectiveness, allows great comfort to serve the patient, for its speed and above all, because the hand makes contact with all the meridians of the body and all its corresponding points. It is also painless. It is comfortable and effective when you have to treat cases of acute pain or trauma. It would be of great importance to experiment with the Churion Detector for diagnosis and treatment.

2- The auriculopuncture.

Auriculotherapy is acupuncture of the ear that is used to activate certain points in the ear which if stimulated correctly, cause a reaction in the nervous system or the area that is sick to achieve the restoration of health. Auriculotherapy has been very effective for weight loss as it helps to avoid fluid retention, decrease appetite and avoid anxiety. It has also been used to treat psychological disorders such as stress and depression. To treat pain, it has been used in neuralgia and sciatica.

The origin of auriculotherapy is quite diffuse in ancient times, by way of summary we will know how auriculopuncture became known in the West. It was the French consul in Beijing George Soulié de Morán who will spread the Traditional Chinese Medicine and with it the auriculotherapy. As a result, the International Society of Acupuncture was formed in Paris in 1927. Then Dr. Paul Nogier released his "Treatise on Auriculotherapy" in 1950.

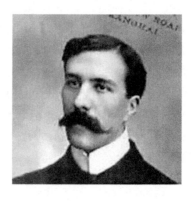

Fig. 29 - George Soulié de Morán. 1878- 1955.

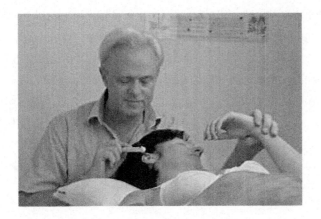

Fig. 30 - Paul Nogier. 1908 – 1996.

3-Diagnosis Method

There are three methods to discover which organ or body part is affected. One of them is visual observation as the appearance of the skin of the ear is a means for the therapist to make certain types of diagnoses. This makes it possible to check the spot and whether there is inflammation. When the color is pale, it may indicate a lack of vitamins and calcium. If the color is red, more or less intense, it indicates kidney problems. If it is too intense, it may be an indication of memory loss, constant headaches and brain problems. As for inflammations, these indicate, according to their

73

intensity, if the disease is chronic or if it is a recent condition. Another method is the manipulation of the ear by which the therapist stimulates various points of the ear until reaching the exact place that is related to the diseased organ. This is checked if the patient feels pain when stimulating the point.

Then, the pain is relieved almost immediately and eventually disappears. But those seconds that the pain lasts are enough for the specialist to identify the affected part. Finally, there is the electronic diagnosis that allows distinguishing, by means of ultrasound waves, the diseased parts from the healthy ones.

Treatment methods. There are several methods of treatment in auriculotherapy:

1- The use of needle
2- The use of seeds
3- The use of magnetic therapy
4- The use of pins
5- The use of micro bleeding
6- The use of moxibustion
7- The use of electrotherapy
8- The use of laser therapy
9- The use of micro massage
10- The use of ultrasound.

Therapeutic index.

This therapeutic index has the particularity that it has to be indicated for only one pathological point, but experience will tell if after performing the treatment with the detector on one point, it can be continued with another, if necessary. For this index we will use the already known points called "The 20 special points" because they allow performing a certain action on tissues, organs and functions. This index may vary with the contributions of acupuncturists.

Abbreviations used to denote the points

BP- Spleen-pancreas meridian.
C- Heart meridian.
Ch- Chamfrault.
CS- Circulation-sexuality meridian.
E- Stomach Meridian.
H- Liver meridian.
Id- Small Intestine meridian.
P- Lung meridian.
R- Kidney meridian.
TR- Meridian of the Triple Superheater.
V- Bladder meridian.
VB- Gallbladder meridian.
VC- Conception vessel.
VG- Governing Vessel.
T- Tonify.
S- Sedate.
Sg- Bleeding.
M- Moxas.

Therapeutic index.

1- Trae-Iuan (9 P): It has action on the circulation of the upper half of the body, especially indicated in hemorrhages.

2- Ro-Kou (4iG): Action on the face, nose, mouth, ears, eyes, pharynx, and teeth. It also has action on the mucous membranes of the digestive tract and the lymphatic system.

3- Tsri-Tchrong (30 E): Stimulates the assimilation of food and sexual functions.

4- Fou-Trou (32): It has action on the peripheral circulation, it is indicated in arterial and venous disorders (intermittent claudication, cooling of the feet, cramps).

5- Sann-Li (36 E): Acts on the general energy, it is indicated in depressive and nervous states.

6- Chang- Tsiou (5 BP): It has action on the connective tissue and venous tone, especially in varicose veins and arthropathies.

7- Sann-Inn. Tsiao (6 BP): It has action on the vascular system and gynecological conditions.

8- Reou-Tsri (3 iD): It has action on water metabolism and sweating. It is very useful in pains and inflammations of all kinds.

9- Tienn-Tchou (10 V): It has action on the parasympathetic.

10- Ta-Tchrou (11 V): Action on the skeletal system, is indicated in spinal disorders and rheumatic joint pain.

11- Ko-Iu (17 V): It is a point of assent of the diaphragm. It has action on blood and circulatory disorders. It is also indicated in all chronic thoracic and abdominal processes.

12- Kao-Roang (38 V): It has action on hematopoiesis. It is indicated in states of weakness: anemia, amenorrhea, weight loss, etc.

13- Oe-Tchong (54 V): It has action on the skin and chronic metabolic disorders, as well as on the lumbar region.

14- Kroun-Loun (60 V): It has action on the states of physical and nervous excitement, in pain of all kinds and in any region, also spasms.

15- Jenn-Kou (2 R): It has action on the adrenal glands, it is indicated in hypertensive states and general excitement.

16- Ling-Siu (24 R): It has action on depressive nervous states, melancholic, related to digestive dysfunctions (Vesicular, gastric, and intestinal).

17- Tchong-Tchrong (9 CS): It has action on vascular tone, it is indicated in hypo and hypertension and arteriosclerosis.

18- Fong-Tchre (20 VB): Action on the sympathetic, is indicated in headaches, insomnia, states of weakness, etc.

19- Iang-Ling-Tsiuan (34 VB): It has action on the muscles.

20- Siuann-Tchong (39 VB): It has action on the nervous system and spinal cord; stimulates leukocytosis; has action on mucosal disorders.

The experience that I have had in analyzing if a person had a discomfort or a pathology in the human body, allowed me to verify that when I analyzed the Ta-Ling source point (7 CS) and I always considered that the person had internal varicose veins, then the patient confirmed it. Another experience that I consider important is that when the Churion Detector is brought close to the ankle on the leg of a person who has abundant amounts of varicose veins, it emits a very strong electrical charge directed towards the handle of the device. In this case, the acupuncturist should grab with the other hand an iron object that is grounded, such as a table or a piece of steel furniture. Afterwards, if he/she considers it, he/she can use the device in the same place.

XII- Medical history.

A clinical history can be provided when the acupuncturists supply us with the information, so that in a second edition of the book we will be able to add them.

APPENDIX

CURE FOR COVID-19 AND DENGUE FEVER WITH A NATURAL MEDICINE

Because of the importance of the cure, because I have been convinced and proven its results. My personal experience comes from the sixties when I was cured of cancer. Then in the eighties I participated in several courses of natural medicine, and published several articles, interviews and reports on the subject. After many experiences with this medicine, it proved to me that it was effective against infections by bacteria, fungi, viruses such as dengue (personal experience) and covid-19. I participated in several medical congresses and my interventions were accepted, then (on one occasion) I had to clarify that I had attended the congress because I was a journalist, not a doctor. In 1995 in an international congress of natural medicine I stepped in presenting my proposal of natural medicine, and when I was going to leave the stage, the assistants began to applaud, and then I had to wait for a long time because the assistants began to stand up and continued applauding.

So, when the covid-19 pandemic started I thought I had a good solution to the issue. I have never charged for the consultations I have done, first because I am not a licensed physician (although I could have done it as a naturopathic doctor) and because my interest has always been to help people without receiving a profit in return.

Diagnosis.

The patient should be asked if he/she suffers from arterial hypertension and also if he/she suffers from HIV-AIDS virus syndrome. In both cases the medicine should not be used.

Preparation of the treatment

A quantity of filtered water is provided; it can be two or three cups. Then calculate the number of cinnamon shells to make a decoction that can take 10 to 15 minutes. It is necessary to be alert to see when the coloration of the water increases, in this way it is verified that the substance that we need to prepare the remedy is released from the shells.

Treatment.

The patient should be given a cup to drink; the effects vary according to the patient: Some feel its effectiveness immediately, others several minutes, and approximately one hour. Then the treatment is continued according to how the patient feels until the definitive cure is achieved.

How does the medication work?

The fact that cinnamon raises blood pressure is due to the fact that in the body there is an increase of white blood cells in the body. This will produce the production of antibodies that will fight the virus present in the human body. When there is an increase in white blood cells, then the body to balance the content of the blood increases the amount of red blood cells, consequently new blood is produced. When a cat is cured, it should be done with a dropper and not give more than one cubic centimeter. I have the bad experience that I recovered the health of a kitten immediately and for giving her a little more, her blood pressure went up and she died immediately. If you have an emergency with a human being that suffers from blood pressure, you can give him/her a small amount, it can be a teaspoon of those that are used to pour sugar in the coffee.

How to perform a scientific test.

Two scientific tests can be performed with cinnamon:
1- A blood test should be performed to determine the amount of white blood cells and red blood cells. After the person has ingested the cinnamon decoction and one hour has passed, a blood test is performed again and the amount of white blood cells is compared with that of the first test; it will

be verified that the amount of white blood cells has increased considerably.

2- You can also use some of the patient's blood that has already been analyzed in the laboratory and place it in a test tube, then add a few drops of the cinnamon decoction, after a certain time has elapsed, it will be verified that the production of white blood cells in the blood contained in the test tube has increased.

How to prepare a natural medicine for mass consumption.

Let's see, aspirin comes from the bark of the white willow tree and cinnamon is also a bark. The inventor of aspirin was the German researcher Felix Hoffman who discovered the remedy in 1897 when he was researching a medicine to cure rheumatoid arthritis suffered by his father? The existing principle in the white willow shell is acetylsalicylic acid, and Hoffman was the first chemist to synthesize it with great purity.

But it is important to note that the first scientist to synthesize acetylsalicylic acid was the French chemist Charles Fréderic Gerhardt in 1853, although he did not synthesize it with great purity.

Aspirin was the commercial name given to Hoffman's discovery by Bayer Laboratories.

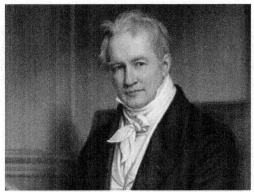

Fig. 31 - Félix Hoffman. 1868 – 1946.

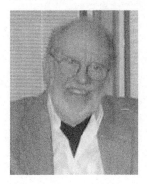

Fig. 32 - Charles Fréderic Gerhardt. 1816 – 1856.

There are two ways to produce a medicine that has its origin in a natural product:

1- One should prepare a decoction of cinnamon and then prepare a syrup that can be bottled in a jar and has a long shelf life for later use.

2- Research should be done using the resources of chemistry to discover the active principle that is found in cinnamon and increases the production of white blood cells in the blood. Perhaps the remedy could be called "Canilin".

Epilogue

Well, now there is the challenge of supplying the Churion Detector. According to the number of requests from interested people, devices will be manufactured. If you are interested in acquiring one, please send all your data to our e-mail.

rjchurion@gmail.com

The other, more important, is the approval of acupuncture in almost all countries of the world. For this purpose, organizations and institutions should ask the United Nations for a congress to discuss the problem. The medical academies should also attend so that they can present their arguments. Finally, a "Modern Acupuncture" should emerge in a definitive way, using all the new resources of physics, electronics and informatics for the benefit of mankind.

Bibliography

B-

Beau, Georges. Acupuncture - Chinese medicine. 1st Edition. Barcelona. Martinez Roca Editions. 1975.

Becker, Robert.O and Gary Selden. The Body Electric- Electromagnetism and the foundation of life. 1st Edition. New York. Quill/105-1985.

Borsarello, Jean. Manual of Acupuncture. 1st Edition Barcelona. Toray Masson. 1982.

C-

Carballo, Floreal. Chinese Acupuncture. 2nd Edition. Buenos Aires. Editorial Kier. 1973.

Carus, Paul. Astrology and Esotericism in China. 1st Edition. Barcelona. Visión Libros, S.L. 1984.

Chin, Ai Li. Psychology in Popular China. 2nd Edition. Bogotá. Editorial Pluma. 1980.

Chuangui, Wang. Chinese Family Acupoint Massage. 3rd Edition. Beijing. Edition. Foreign language editions. 1995.

Chenggu, Ye. Treatment of Mental Illness by acupuncture and moxibustion. 1st Edition. Beijing. Foreign language editions. 1992.

Crèpon, Pierre. Practical dictionary of acupuncture and acupressure. 1st Edition. Bilbao. Ediciones Mensajero. 1982.

Conghuo, Tian. 101 diseases treated with Acupuncture and Moxibustion. 1st Edition. Beijing. Foreign language editions. 1992.

D-

Duke, Marc. Acupuncture- The Chinese art of healing. 1st Edition. Barcelona. Bella Terra Editions. 1973.

De Marre, Dean.A and David Michaels. Bioelectronic Measurements. 1st Edition. New Jersey. Prentice Hall.1983.

G-

Guillén, Vicente. Practical Manual of Auriculotherapy and Acupuncture. 1st Edition. Barcelona. Ediciones Teorema. 1985.

I- Hispanic Institute of Acupuncture. Vademecum of Auriculotherapy. 1st Edition. Madrid. Ediciones Miraguano. 1986.

K-

Kiang, Yang Tse. Acupuncture. 1st Edition. Buenos Aires. Editorial Albatros. 1975.

L-

Lawson, Denis. W and Joyce L. W. The Five Elements of Acupuncture and Chinese Massage. 1st Edition. Venezuela. Barnaven. 1988.

M-

Mehta, Anil. K. Magnetotherapy and acupuncture. 1st Edition. Buenos Aires. Ediciones Continente. 1994.

N-

Nian, Shao Fang. Diagnostics of Traditional Chinese Medicine. 1st Edition. Beijing. Shandong Science and Technology. 1990.

Nogier, Paul. Auriculotherapy. Auriculomedicine. 1st Edition. Buenos Aires. Editorial Albastros. 1992.

P-

Pinto, C. Mishaan. Acupuncture - Science or charlatanism. 1st Edition. Barcelona. Ediciones Bellaterra. 1980.

S-

Sussmann, David. J. ACUPUNCTURE- Theory and practice. 13th edition. Buenos Aires. Editorial Kier. 2000.

Scott, Pauline.M. Electrotherapy and Actinotherapy. 1st Edition. Barcelona. Editorial JIMS. 1972.

Z-

Zhengguang, Chen. The Orthopedic Treatment of Traditional Chinese Medicine. 1st Edition. Beijing. Foreign Language Editions. 1992.

W-

Wallnofer, Heinrich and Anna von R. All Chinese Healing Methods. 1st Edition. Barcelona. Martinez Roca Editions. 1980.

Weikang, Fu. Acupuncture and Moxibustion- Historical outline. 1st Edition. Foreign language editions. 1983.

Other works by the author

Introduction to Modern Dowsing

Mental Power Techniques: Trough Modern Radiesthesia

Contact with the author.

Users who have used this work and would like to contribute with knowledge or experience are welcome. If you would like to purchase the Churion Detector please send us your details and we will get back to you as soon as possible.

E-mail us: rjchurion@gmail.com

Printed in Great Britain
by Amazon

40842442R00050